Diabetes Healthy lifestyle

Achieving Optimal Health with Diabetes.

George G. Bissett

Disclaimer

This document contains proprietary information
and intellectual property belonging to GeorgeG.
Bissett. Any unauthorized use or disclosure of
this information is prohibited.

George G. Bissett reserves the right to make
changes to the content of this document at any
time without prior notice.

Table of Contents

Introduction

Grace had always struggled with her weight and health. Despite her best efforts, she had been unable to shake the extra pounds that seemed to cling to her no matter what she did. She had always been a bit self-conscious about her appearance, but it wasn't until she was diagnosed with diabetes that she really began to worry.

At first, Grace was devastated by the news. She had always known that her unhealthy habits were catching up with her, but she had never imagined that she would be faced with such a serious condition. She was terrified at the thought of having to inject herself with insulin every day or suffer the consequences of uncontrolled blood sugar levels.

But Grace was determined not to let her diabetes defeat her. She made the decision to take control of her health and do whatever it took to get her condition under control. With the help of this book and a nutritionist, she began making major changes to her diet.

Gone were the processed foods and sugary snacks that had always been a staple of her diet. In their place, Grace began incorporating more fruits, vegetables, and whole grains into her meals. She also made an effort to get more physical activity, going for daily walks and eventually joining a gym.

The changes didn't come easy for Grace, but she was determined to stick with them. And after just a few months, she began to see real results. Her blood sugar levels were steadily improving, and she was starting to feel better than she had in years.

As the months passed, Grace's diabetes went into full remission. She was able to stop taking insulin altogether, and her overall health had improved dramatically. She had finally achieved the healthy weight and active lifestyle that she had always wanted, and it was all thanks to the right diet and lifestyle changes.

Grace was thrilled with her success and couldn't believe how much her life had changed. She had always thought that diabetes was a death sentence, but she had proved that with the right mindset and determination, anything was possible.

Chapter One

What is diabetes and how does it affect the body?

Diabetes is a chronic medical condition that affects the way the body processes blood sugar (glucose). Glucose is a type of sugar that is the body's main source of energy. In order for glucose to be used as energy, it needs to be transported from the bloodstream into cells. This process is regulated by a hormone called insulin, which is produced by the pancreas.

There are two main types of diabetes: type 1 and type 2.

Type 1 diabetes is an autoimmune disorder in which the body's immune system attacks and destroys the cells in the pancreas that produce insulin. This means that people with type 1 diabetes do not produce any insulin and must take insulin injections or use an insulin pump to regulate their blood sugar. Type 1 diabetes is usually diagnosed in children and young adults, although it can occur at any age.

Type 2 diabetes is a metabolic disorder that occurs when the body becomes resistant to insulin or when the pancreas is unable to produce enough insulin to meet the body's needs. This can cause the body's blood sugar levels to become too high. Type 2 diabetes is the most common form of diabetes and is often linked to being overweight or obese, having a sedentary lifestyle, and having a family history of diabetes.

Both types of diabetes can lead to serious health problems if left untreated. High blood sugar levels can damage the blood vessels and nerves, leading to problems such as heart disease, stroke, kidney disease, blindness, and nerve damage. Diabetes can also increase the risk of developing certain types of cancer.

To manage diabetes, people with the condition may need to make lifestyle changes, such as eating a healthy diet, getting regular physical activity, and maintaining a healthy weight. They may also need to take medications or insulin injections to help regulate their blood sugar levels. By carefully managing their diabetes, people with the condition can often lead healthy, active lives.

☐ The role of diet and lifestyle in managing diabetes

Diet and lifestyle play a crucial role in managing diabetes. A healthy diet and regular physical activity can help to control blood sugar levels and prevent complications from diabetes.

Here are some specific ways that diet and lifestyle can help manage diabetes:

- **Maintaining a balanced diet:** A balanced diet for people with diabetes should include a variety of nutrient-dense foods such as fruits, vegetables, whole grains, and lean proteins. It is also important to limit intake of added sugars and saturated fats.

- **Monitoring carbohydrate intake:** Carbohydrates are a major source of energy, but they can also affect blood sugar levels. People with diabetes should aim to eat a consistent amount of carbohydrates at each meal and snack. This can be achieved by counting carbs or using exchange lists.

- **Incorporating physical activity:** Physical activity can help lower blood sugar levels and improve insulin sensitivity. It is recommended that people with diabetes get at least 150 minutes of moderate-intensity aerobic activity per week.

- **Managing stress:** Chronic stress can lead to unhealthy behaviors, such as overeating and lack of physical activity, which can affect blood sugar control. It is important for people with diabetes to find ways to manage stress, such as through relaxation techniques, exercise, or seeking support from friends and family.

- **Quitting smoking:** Smoking increases the risk of complications from diabetes, such as heart disease and nerve damage. Quitting smoking can help improve blood sugar control and reduce the risk of complications.

In summary, a healthy diet, regular physical activity, and managing stress and unhealthy habits can all play a role in helping to manage diabetes. It is important to work with a healthcare team, including a doctor and a registered dietitian, to develop a plan that works for individual needs and preferences.

Chapter Two

Understanding carbohydrates and blood sugar

Carbohydrates are an important source of energy for the body and can be found in a variety of foods, including grains, fruits, vegetables, and dairy products. When you eat carbohydrates, your body converts them into glucose, which is absorbed into the bloodstream. As the level of glucose in your blood increases, your pancreas releases the hormone insulin, which helps your cells to use the glucose for energy.

There are two main types of carbohydrates: simple and complex. Simple carbohydrates are found in foods that are easily broken down by the body and include things like sugar, honey, and fruit. They are quickly absorbed into the bloodstream, which can cause a rapid increase in blood sugar levels.

Complex carbohydrates, on the other hand, are found in foods like grains, beans, and vegetables. They are made up of long chains of glucose and take longer to digest and be absorbed into the bloodstream. This means that they can help to provide a slower, more sustained release of energy and can help to regulate blood sugar levels.

In general, it's important to include a variety of carbohydrates in your diet, as they provide energy and nutrients that your body needs to function properly. However, it's also important to be mindful of the amount and type of carbohydrates that you are consuming, as this can affect your blood sugar levels.

Here are a few tips for managing blood sugar levels through your diet:

- Choose complex carbohydrates over simple carbohydrates whenever possible.

- Eat a variety of fruits, vegetables, and whole grains to ensure that you are getting a variety of nutrients.

- Control portion sizes, as eating too much of any type of carbohydrate can cause a rapid increase in blood sugar.

- Eat protein and healthy fats with carbohydrates to help slow down the absorption of glucose into the bloodstream.

Consider the glycemic index (GI) of the foods you are eating. The GI is a measure of how quickly a food is likely to raise your blood sugar levels. Foods with a high GI (like white bread and sugary drinks) are absorbed quickly and can cause a rapid increase in blood sugar. Foods with a low GI (like whole grains and most vegetables) are absorbed more slowly and can help to regulate blood sugar levels.

It's important to maintain healthy blood sugar levels, as high or low blood sugar can have negative health effects. High blood sugar, or hyperglycemia, can occur if the body is not producing enough insulin or if the cells are not responding properly to insulin. This can lead to long-term complications such as nerve damage, blindness, and kidney disease. On the other hand, low blood sugar, or hypoglycemia, can occur if you have taken too much insulin or other medications, or if you have not eaten enough food. This can cause symptoms such as dizziness, sweating, and shaking.

Remember that everyone is different and what works for one person may not work for another. It's important to work with a healthcare professional to determine the best approach for managing your blood sugar levels.

☐ **How carbohydrates affect blood sugar levels**

Carbohydrates are an important source of energy for the body and can be found in a variety of foods, including grains, fruits, vegetables, and dairy products. When you eat carbohydrates, your body converts them into glucose, which is absorbed into the bloodstream. As the level of glucose in your blood increases, your pancreas releases the hormone insulin, which helps your cells to use the glucose for energy.

Eating a balanced diet that includes a variety of carbohydrates, such as whole grains, fruits, and vegetables, can help to maintain healthy blood sugar levels. It's important to choose complex carbohydrates, which are high in fiber and tend to be digested more slowly, rather than simple carbohydrates, which are quickly absorbed into the bloodstream. This can help to prevent rapid fluctuations in blood sugar levels.

Physical activity can also help to regulate blood sugar levels by increasing the body's sensitivity to insulin and helping to move glucose out of the bloodstream and into the cells. Regular exercise can also help to improve the overall function of the body's cells and tissues, which can further support healthy blood sugar management.

It's important to maintain healthy blood sugar levels, as high or low blood sugar can have negative health effects. High blood sugar, or hyperglycemia, can occur if the body is not producing enough insulin or if the cells are not responding properly to insulin. This can lead to long-term complications such as nerve damage, blindness, and kidney disease. On the other hand, low blood sugar, or hypoglycemia, can occur if you have taken too much insulin or other medications, or if you have not eaten enough food. This can cause symptoms such as dizziness, sweating, and shaking.

If you have a condition such as diabetes, it is important to work with a healthcare team to manage your blood sugar levels through a combination of medication, diet, and physical activity. Regular monitoring of your blood sugar levels can help to identify any issues and allow for adjustments to your treatment plan as needed

☐ **Choosing the right types of carbohydrates**

For people with diabetes, it's important to choose carbohydrates that are balanced with protein and healthy fats to help regulate blood sugar levels. Here are some tips for choosing the right types of carbohydrates as a person with diabetes:

- Focus on whole grains and fiber-rich carbs: Whole grains and foods high in fiber, such as vegetables and legumes, can help slow the absorption of glucose into the bloodstream and help regulate blood sugar levels.

- Watch portion sizes: It's important to pay attention to portion sizes, especially for high-carb foods, to avoid spikes in blood sugar. A registered dietitian or certified diabetes educator can help you determine the right portion sizes for your needs.

- Choose healthy fats: Adding healthy fats, such as those found in avocados, nuts, and olive oil, to meals and snacks can help slow the absorption of carbohydrates and improve blood sugar control.

- Consider the glycemic index (GI): The glycemic index is a ranking of carbohydrates based on how they affect blood sugar levels. Foods with a low GI (less than 55) are absorbed more slowly and can help regulate blood sugar levels, while foods with a high GI (greater than 70) are absorbed more quickly and can cause spikes in blood sugar.

Chapter Three

The diabetes reversal diet

The diabetes reversal diet is a dietary approach that focuses on making changes to the types and amounts of carbohydrates, fats, and proteins consumed in order to improve blood sugar control and potentially reverse type 2 diabetes. This approach typically involves reducing the intake of refined carbohydrates, added sugars, and unhealthy fats, and increasing the intake of whole grains, vegetables, and healthy fats.

Some people may also choose to follow a low-carbohydrate diet or a vegan diet, as these approaches have been shown to improve blood sugar control in some individuals.

Some key components of the diabetes reversal diet include:

1. **Increasing fiber intake:** Foods high in fiber, such as vegetables, whole grains, and legumes, can help slow the absorption of glucose into the bloodstream and improve blood sugar control.

2. **Reducing intake of added sugars:** Added sugars, such as those found in sweetened beverages and processed foods, can contribute empty calories to the diet and increase the risk of insulin resistance and other health problems. Limiting added sugars can help improve blood sugar control.

3. **Increasing intake of healthy fats:** Healthy fats, such as those found in

avocados, nuts, and olive oil, can help improve blood sugar control and reduce the risk of heart disease.

4. **Incorporating physical activity:** Regular physical activity can help improve insulin sensitivity and blood sugar control, and can be an important part of a diabetes reversal plan.

It's important to note that the diabetes reversal diet should be customized to an individual's specific needs and should be followed under the guidance of a healthcare professional. While some people with type 2 diabetes may be able to achieve full reversal, others may need to continue taking medications even if they make dietary and lifestyle changes.

Overall, the diabetes reversal diet can be a helpful tool for improving blood sugar control and overall health in some individuals with diabetes, but it's important to work with a healthcare professional to determine the best approach for your individual needs.

☐ Understanding portion sizes and calorie needs

Portion sizes refer to the amount of a particular food that you choose to eat, while calorie needs refer to the number of calories that your body requires to fuel your daily activities. The appropriate portion size and calorie needs can vary based on a variety of factors, including your age, gender, weight, height, and physical activity level.

To determine your calorie needs, you can use an online calculator or consult with a healthcare professional. There are also general guidelines that can provide a rough estimate of your calorie needs. For example, adult men generally require more calories than adult women, and physically active people generally require more calories than sedentary people.

In general, it is recommended to aim for a balanced diet that includes a variety of nutrient-dense foods in appropriate portion sizes. This can help you meet your nutrient needs and maintain a healthy weight. It is also important to pay attention to portion sizes, as consuming too many calories can lead to weight gain, while consuming too few calories can lead to malnutrition.

To help you understand portion sizes and make healthier choices, here are some general guidelines for common foods:

1 serving of fruit is about the size of a tennis ball
1 serving of vegetables is about the size of a fist

1 serving of grains is about the size of a baseball

1 serving of meat is about the size of a deck of cards

1 serving of nuts is about the size of a small handful

Remember that these are just general guidelines and that portion sizes can vary based on your individual calorie needs. It is always a good idea to pay attention to the serving size listed on food labels and to be mindful of how much you are consuming.

Chapter Four

Incorporating healthy fats, proteins, and non-starchy vegetables

Eating a diet that includes healthy fats, proteins, and non-starchy vegetables is important for maintaining overall health and well-being. These nutrients can help to support a variety of bodily functions and provide the energy and nutrients needed to maintain good health. Here are some tips for incorporating these nutrients into your diet:

- **Include healthy fats:** Healthy fats, such as olive oil, avocado, nuts, and seeds, are an important part of a healthy diet. They provide energy and support the absorption of certain vitamins and minerals. Try using olive oil when cooking, adding avocado to sandwiches and salads, and snacking on a handful of nuts or seeds.

- **Choose high-protein foods:** Protein is essential for building and repairing tissues, producing enzymes and hormones, and helping to maintain fluid balance. Good sources of protein include poultry, seafood, beans, nuts, and tofu. Try adding chicken, fish, or tofu to your meals, or incorporating beans and nuts into your snacks.

- **Eat plenty of non-starchy vegetables:** Non-starchy vegetables, such as leafy greens, broccoli, bell peppers, and cucumbers, are low in calories and high in fiber, vitamins, and minerals. They can help to fill you up and keep you feeling satisfied, making it easier to maintain a healthy weight. Try adding a variety of non-starchy vegetables to your meals and snacks, and aim for at least 5 servings a day.

By incorporating these healthy fats, proteins, and non-starchy vegetables into your diet, you can ensure that you're getting the nutrients you need to stay healthy and feel your best.

☐ **Meal planning and recipe ideas for diabetes**

Eating a healthy, balanced diet is important for everyone, but it's especially important for people with diabetes to manage their blood sugar levels. Here are a few tips for meal planning and finding recipe ideas for diabetes:

1. **Focus on whole, unprocessed foods:** Choose foods that are minimally processed, such as fresh fruits and vegetables, whole grains, lean proteins, and healthy fats.

2. **Include a variety of nutrients:** Make sure to get a mix of nutrients in your meals, including protein, fiber, healthy fats, and complex carbs.

3. **Plan ahead:** Meal planning can help you stay on track and make healthier choices. Try to plan your meals and snacks in advance, and keep healthy options on hand for when you're short on time.

4. **Keep an eye on portion sizes:** It's important to pay attention to portion sizes, especially when it comes to carbohydrates. Use measuring cups or a kitchen scale to help you get an accurate idea of how much you're eating.

5. **Don't forget about physical activity:** Regular physical activity can help you manage your blood sugar levels and improve your overall health. Try to incorporate at least 30 minutes of moderate-intensity activity into your daily routine.

Here are a few recipe ideas to get you started:

Breakfast Recipes

Overnight Oats with Blueberries and Almonds: Combine 1/2 cup old-fashioned oats, 1/2 cup unsweetened almond milk, 1/2 cup fresh or frozen blueberries, and 1 tablespoon chopped almonds in a jar or container. Cover and refrigerate overnight. In the morning, top with a sprinkle of cinnamon and a drizzle of honey or maple syrup, if desired.

Egg and Vegetable Breakfast Wrap: Heat a small amount of olive oil in a pan over medium heat. Add 1/2 cup chopped vegetables (such as bell peppers, onions, and mushrooms) and cook until tender. Crack 2 eggs into the pan and scramble until fully cooked. Place the eggs and vegetables in a whole wheat tortilla, along with 1/4 cup shredded cheese and a few leaves of fresh spinach. Roll up the tortilla and enjoy.

Greek Yogurt Parfait: In a jar or glass, layer 1/2 cup plain Greek yogurt, 1/4 cup granola, and 1/2 cup sliced fresh fruit (such as berries, banana, or kiwi). Repeat the layers once more, then top with a sprinkle of chia seeds and a drizzle of honey or maple syrup, if desired.

Avocado Toast with Egg: Toast 1 slice of whole grain bread until crispy. Mash 1/4 of an avocado onto the toast, then top with a fried or poached egg. Season with a pinch of salt and pepper, and enjoy.

Breakfast Smoothie Bowl: In a blender, combine 1/2 cup unsweetened almond milk, 1/2 banana, 1/4 cup frozen berries, 1/4 cup spinach, 1 scoop protein powder, and a few ice cubes. Blend until smooth. Pour the smoothie into a bowl and top with a sprinkle of chia seeds, a few slices of banana, and a tablespoon of chopped nuts.

Lunch Recipes

Quinoa and Black Bean Salad: Cook quinoa according to package instructions and set aside to cool. In a separate pan, sauté diced bell peppers, onions, and black beans until tender. Mix the cooled quinoa, sautéed vegetables, and a can of drained and rinsed black beans in a large bowl. Add in a handful of chopped fresh cilantro and a squeeze of lime juice. Top with diced avocado and serve.

Turkey and Veggie Wrap: Spread a whole grain tortilla with hummus and top with sliced turkey, shredded lettuce, sliced tomato, and grated carrot. Roll up the tortilla and slice in half to serve.

Grilled Chicken and Roasted Vegetable Salad: Grill a chicken breast until cooked through and slice into thin strips. Toss sliced chicken with roasted vegetables (such as bell peppers, onions, and zucchini) and a handful of mixed greens. Top with a homemade vinaigrette dressing made with olive oil, red wine vinegar, and a pinch of dijon mustard.

Salmon and Quinoa Bowl: Cook quinoa according to package instructions and set aside. Meanwhile, bake a salmon fillet until cooked through. Assemble the bowl by placing the quinoa in the bottom, followed by the salmon, steamed broccoli, and a sprinkle of sliced almonds. Top with a homemade lemon tahini dressing made with tahini, lemon juice, and water.

Egg and Avocado Toast: Toast a slice of whole grain bread until crispy. Top with mashed avocado and a fried egg. Season with salt and pepper to taste. Serve with a side of mixed fruit.

Dinner Recipes

Grilled Chicken and Vegetable Skewers: Thread bite-sized pieces of chicken and vegetables (such as bell peppers, onions, and zucchini) onto skewers. Grill until the chicken is cooked through and the vegetables are tender. Serve with a side of quinoa or brown rice.

Spaghetti Squash with Turkey Meatballs: Cut a spaghetti squash in half and remove the seeds. Place the squash, cut-side down, in a baking dish and roast in the oven until tender. Meanwhile, mix ground turkey, diced onion, minced garlic, and a few tablespoons of breadcrumbs to make meatballs. Brown the meatballs in a pan on the stove and set aside. When the squash is tender, use a fork to scrape out the strands and place them in a large bowl. Add the meatballs to the bowl and top with a homemade tomato sauce made with diced tomatoes, garlic, and basil.

Salmon and Roasted Vegetable Quinoa Bowl: Cook quinoa according to package instructions and set aside. Meanwhile, roast a selection of vegetables (such as bell peppers, onions, and zucchini) in the oven until tender. Top the quinoa with the roasted vegetables and a baked salmon fillet. Serve with a side of steamed broccoli.

Chili: In a large pot, sauté diced onions, bell peppers, and minced garlic in a bit of oil until tender. Add in ground turkey and cook until browned. Stir in a can of diced tomatoes, a can of kidney beans (drained and rinsed), and a few tablespoons of chili powder. Bring the mixture to a boil, then reduce the heat and simmer for 10-15 minutes. Serve with a side of brown rice or quinoa.

Baked Chicken and Sweet Potato: Preheat the oven to 400°F. Place a chicken breast and a peeled and diced sweet potato on a baking sheet.

Season with a bit of olive oil, salt, and pepper and roast until the chicken is cooked through and the sweet potato is tender. Serve with a side of steamed broccoli.

Remember, it's important to work with a healthcare professional to come up with a meal plan that's right for you and your individual needs. They can help you develop healthy eating habits and provide guidance on how to manage your blood sugar levels.

Chapter Five

Lifestyle changes for diabetes reversal

Making lifestyle changes is an important part of managing and reversing diabetes. Here are some steps you can take to improve your health and manage your diabetes:

1. Eat a healthy diet: Choose foods that are low in added sugars, saturated and trans fats, and sodium, and focus on eating whole, unprocessed foods like fruits, vegetables, whole grains, lean proteins, and healthy fats.

2. Get regular physical activity: Aim for at least 30 minutes of moderate-intensity exercise, such as brisk walking or cycling, on most days of the week. This can help improve insulin sensitivity and lower blood sugar levels.

3. Lose weight: If you are overweight or obese, losing weight can help improve your blood sugar control and decrease your risk of diabetes complications. Aim for a slow, steady weight loss of about 1 to 2 pounds per week by eating a healthy diet and getting regular physical activity.

4. Manage stress: Stress can cause blood sugar levels to rise, so it's important to find healthy ways to manage stress, such as through relaxation techniques, exercise, or talking to a therapist.

5. Quit smoking: Smoking can increase your risk of diabetes complications, such as heart disease and nerve damage. If you smoke, quitting can help improve your overall health and lower your risk of complications.

6. Get enough sleep: Getting enough sleep is important for maintaining good blood sugar

control. Aim for 7 to 9 hours of sleep per night.

7. Monitor your blood sugar levels: Regular blood sugar monitoring can help you and your healthcare team determine the effectiveness of your treatment plan and make any necessary adjustments.

It's important to work with a healthcare team, including a doctor, dietitian, and possibly a diabetes educator, to develop a treatment plan that works for you.

It's also worth noting that reversing diabetes is not always possible, and the potential for reversal may depend on the type of diabetes and the length of time the individual has had diabetes. However, making lifestyle changes can still be beneficial for improving blood sugar control and reducing the risk of complications from diabetes.

Making lifestyle changes can be challenging, but with the right support and guidance, you can make lasting changes that can help improve your health and reverse your diabetes.

☐ **Exercise and physical activity for diabetes reversal**

Exercise and physical activity can be an important part of managing and reversing diabetes. Regular physical activity can help improve insulin sensitivity, lower blood sugar levels, and reduce the risk of complications associated with diabetes. It can also help with weight loss, which can further improve insulin sensitivity and blood sugar control.

Here are some tips for incorporating exercise into your routine if you have diabetes:

- Consult with your healthcare provider before starting a new exercise routine, especially if you have any underlying health conditions.

- Start slowly and gradually increase the intensity and duration of your workouts over time. Aim for at least 150 minutes of moderate-intensity aerobic exercise per week, or at least 75 minutes of vigorous-intensity aerobic exercise per week. This can be broken down into shorter periods of activity throughout the week.

- Include strength training exercises at least two days per week to help improve muscle strength and insulin sensitivity. Choose activities that you enjoy and that are convenient for your lifestyle. Some examples include walking, swimming, cycling, dancing, and yoga.

- Monitor your blood sugar levels before and after exercise to see how it affects your levels and make adjustments as needed.

- Stay hydrated by drinking water before, during, and after your workouts.

It's important to remember that while exercise can be an important part of managing and reversing diabetes, it's just one piece of the puzzle. A healthy diet, stress management techniques, and regular medical care are also important for managing and reversing diabetes

☐ **Stress management and relaxation techniques**

There are several stress management and relaxation techniques that may be helpful in managing diabetes and potentially reversing the disease:

1. Exercise: Regular physical activity can help reduce stress and improve blood sugar control.

2. Meditation and mindfulness: These practices involve focusing your attention on the present moment and letting go of distracting thoughts. They can help you relax and manage stress.

3. Deep breathing: Taking slow, deep breaths can help you relax and reduce stress.

4. Progressive muscle relaxation: This technique involves tensing and relaxing different muscle groups to promote relaxation.

5. Yoga: This physical and mental discipline involves various postures and breathing techniques that can help reduce stress and improve overall health.

6. Massage: Massage can help reduce stress and improve circulation, which can be beneficial for people with diabetes.

7. Acupuncture: This traditional Chinese medicine technique involves inserting thin needles into specific points on the body to promote relaxation and improve overall health.

It's important to note that while these techniques may be helpful in managing stress and improving overall health, they should not be used as a replacement for medical treatment for diabetes. It's important to work with a healthcare professional to create a treatment plan that is appropriate for your individual needs.

☐ **Sleep and sleep hygiene**

Maintaining healthy sleep habits can be beneficial for people with diabetes, as well as those who are trying to reverse the condition. Here are some tips for improving sleep hygiene in the context of diabetes:

- Stick to a consistent sleep schedule: Try to go to bed and wake up at the same time every day, even on weekends. This can help regulate your body's natural sleep-wake cycle.

- Create a relaxing bedtime routine: Wind down before bed by engaging in activities such as reading, taking a warm bath, or listening to soothing music.

- Make your sleep environment comfortable: Keep your bedroom cool, dark, and quiet, and use a comfortable mattress and pillows.

- Avoid caffeine, alcohol, and large meals close to bedtime: These can disrupt your sleep.

- Avoid screens before bed: The blue light emitted by electronic devices can disrupt your natural sleep patterns. Consider using a screen filter or setting a bedtime for your devices.

- Exercise during the day: Regular physical activity can help improve sleep quality. Just be sure to finish your workout a few hours before bed so your body has time to wind down.

- Manage stress: Stress and anxiety can interfere with sleep. Consider trying relaxation techniques such as deep breathing or meditation to help you relax before bed.

By following these tips and working with a healthcare professional, you can improve your sleep hygiene and potentially support your efforts to reverse diabetes. It's important to note that while making lifestyle changes can be beneficial, diabetes reversal is not always possible and may require medical treatment.

Chapter Six

Supplements and medications

It is important to note that there is currently no known cure for diabetes and no supplements or medications that have been proven to reverse the condition. Diabetes is a chronic disease that requires ongoing medical management and lifestyle changes to help manage blood sugar levels and prevent complications.

While some supplements and medications may be used to help manage blood sugar levels in people with diabetes, they are not a cure for the condition. It is important to work with a healthcare provider to develop a treatment plan that is right for you and to follow your treatment plan as directed. This may include taking medications, making lifestyle changes (such as eating a healthy diet and getting regular physical activity), and monitoring blood sugar levels regularly.

Medications:

Insulin: This hormone is produced by the pancreas and is necessary for the body to use glucose for energy. People with type 1 diabetes and some people with type 2 diabetes may need to take insulin injections or use an insulin pump to help regulate their blood sugar levels.

Oral medications: There are several types of oral medications that can be used to help control blood sugar levels in people with type 2 diabetes. These medications work by increasing the production of insulin, decreasing the amount of glucose produced by the liver, or helping the body use insulin more effectively.

Supplements:

Chromium: Some research suggests that chromium supplements may help improve blood sugar control in people with type 2 diabetes. However, more research is needed to confirm this.

Alpha-lipoic acid: This antioxidant has been suggested as a potential treatment for diabetes, but there is limited scientific evidence to support its use.

Some people with type 2 diabetes may be able to achieve partial or complete remission of their diabetes through weight loss and lifestyle changes, but this is not the same as a cure and the diabetes is likely to return if the individual returns to their previous lifestyle.

It is important to speak with a healthcare provider before starting any new supplement or medication regimen, as some supplements and medications can interact with each other or with other conditions you may have. Additionally, self-treating diabetes with supplements or medications without proper medical supervision can be dangerous.

☐ The role of supplements in diabetes management

Supplements may be used as part of a diabetes management plan in some cases, but they should not be used as a replacement for a healthy diet and regular physical activity. It is important to speak with a healthcare provider before starting any new supplement regimen, as some supplements can interact with medications or other conditions you may have.

Some supplements that have been suggested as potentially helpful in managing diabetes include chromium, alpha-lipoic acid, and magnesium.

Chromium: Some research suggests that chromium supplements may help improve blood sugar control in people with type 2 diabetes, but more research is needed to confirm this.

Alpha-lipoic acid: This antioxidant has been suggested as a potential treatment for diabetes, but there is limited scientific evidence to support its use.

However, the evidence supporting the use of these supplements for the treatment of diabetes is limited, and more research is needed to fully understand their effectiveness.

It is important to note that supplements are not regulated by the Food and Drug Administration (FDA) in the same way that medications are, and the quality and purity of supplements can vary widely. This means that it is important to be cautious when using supplements and to choose products from reputable manufacturers.

Overall, the most effective way to manage diabetes is to work with a healthcare provider to develop a comprehensive treatment plan that includes medications (if necessary), lifestyle changes, and regular monitoring of blood sugar levels.

☐ Working with a healthcare provider to adjust medication doses

It is important to work closely with a healthcare provider to manage diabetes and adjust medication doses as needed. Diabetes is a chronic condition that requires ongoing medical attention and management to prevent complications. If you are taking medication to manage your diabetes, it is important to follow your healthcare provider's instructions and take your medication as directed. If you have any questions or concerns about your medication or treatment plan, be sure to discuss them with your healthcare provider. They can help you understand your treatment options and make any necessary adjustments to your medication doses to help you better manage your diabetes.

Here are some things you can do to help:

1. Keep track of your blood sugar levels: Regularly testing your blood sugar levels can help your healthcare provider understand how well your current treatment plan is working and make any necessary adjustments.

2. Follow your treatment plan: Make sure to take your medications as prescribed and follow any other recommendations from your healthcare provider, such as following a healthy diet and getting regular exercise.

3. Communicate with your healthcare provider: If you have any concerns or questions about your treatment plan, don't

hesitate to bring them up with your healthcare provider. They can help address your concerns and make any necessary adjustments.

4. Be proactive: If you notice any changes in your blood sugar levels or if you experience any side effects from your medications, let your healthcare provider know right away. This can help them make adjustments to your treatment plan to ensure that it is as effective as possible.

It's important to remember that managing diabetes requires ongoing care and attention. By working closely with your healthcare provider and following their recommendations, you can help ensure that your treatment plan is as effective as possible in controlling your blood sugar levels and helping you live a healthy, active life.

Chapter Seven

Managing Diabetes in the long term

Managing diabetes in the long term requires a combination of lifestyle changes, medication, and regular medical care. Some things you can do to help manage your diabetes in the long term include:

Follow a healthy dict: This typically involves eating a variety of nutritious foods in appropriate portions, such as fruits, vegetables, whole grains, and lean proteins. Your healthcare provider or a registered dietitian can help you develop a meal plan that meets your individual needs.

Get regular exercise: Regular physical activity can help you manage your blood sugar levels, maintain a healthy weight, and reduce your risk of complications. Aim for at least 30 minutes of moderate-intensity exercise, such as brisk walking, most days of the week.

Take your medications as prescribed: It's important to follow your treatment plan as prescribed by your healthcare provider. This may include taking medications to control your blood sugar levels and prevent complications.

Monitor your blood sugar levels: Regularly testing your blood sugar levels can help you and your healthcare provider understand how well your treatment plan is working and make any necessary adjustments.

Attend regular medical appointments: It's important to see your healthcare provider regularly to monitor your diabetes and manage any complications. They may also recommend additional tests, such as a hemoglobin A1c test, to check your blood sugar control over the past two to three months.

By following these recommendations and working closely with your healthcare provider, you can help effectively manage your diabetes in the long term and reduce your risk of complications.

☐ **Continuing to make healthy lifestyle choices**

Continuing to make healthy lifestyle choices is important for maintaining good health and managing chronic conditions such as diabetes. Here are some tips for making and maintaining healthy lifestyle changes:

Set specific, achievable goals: Make a plan and set specific goals for yourself, such as eating a certain number of servings of fruits and vegetables per day or exercising for a certain amount of time each week.

Track your progress: Use a journal or a tracking app to keep track of your progress. This can help you stay motivated and identify areas where you may need to make additional changes.

Seek support: Consider enlisting the support of friends, family, or a healthcare professional to help you stay on track.

Don't be too hard on yourself: It's normal to have setbacks and make mistakes. Don't let a slip-up discourage you from continuing to make healthy choices.

Find healthy ways to cope with stress: Chronic stress can affect your blood sugar levels and your overall health. Find healthy ways to cope with stress, such as through relaxation techniques or talking to a therapist.

By making and maintaining healthy lifestyle choices, you can improve your blood sugar control, reduce your risk of complications, and maintain good overall health. It's important to work with your healthcare team to develop a plan that works for you.

☐ **Monitoring blood sugar levels and adjusting the plan as needed.**

Monitoring blood sugar levels and adjusting the plan as needed is an important aspect of diabetes management. There are several ways to monitor blood sugar levels, including:

Self-monitoring of blood glucose (SMBG): This involves using a blood glucose meter to measure your blood sugar levels at home. You will need to prick your finger to obtain a small drop of blood, which you will then apply to a test strip that is inserted into the meter. The meter will give you a reading of your blood sugar level in milligrams per deciliter (mg/dL).

Continuous glucose monitoring (CGM): This involves wearing a small device that continuously measures your blood sugar levels and sends the data to a device, such as a smartphone, that you can view.

HbA1c test: This test measures your average blood sugar level over the past 2-3 months. It is typically done in a lab or at your doctor's office and does not require you to fast or stop taking your medications.

It's important to work with a healthcare team, including a primary care doctor, endocrinologist, and possibly a diabetes educator, to develop a plan for monitoring your blood sugar levels and adjusting your treatment plan as needed. This may involve making changes to your diet, physical activity, and medications. It's also important to regularly review your blood sugar levels with your healthcare team to assess how well your treatment plan is working and make any necessary adjustments.

☐ Coping with setbacks and maintaining motivation

Managing diabetes can be challenging, and it is common for people to experience setbacks or challenges along the way. It is important to remember that it is normal to have ups and downs, and that it is okay to ask for help when you need it. Here are some strategies for coping with setbacks and maintaining motivation:

1. Seek support: Talk to your healthcare team, friends, and family about your challenges and how they can support you. Consider joining a support group for people with diabetes, which can provide a

sense of community and help you feel less alone.

2. Set realistic goals: Setting goals that are too ambitious can lead to disappointment and frustration. Instead, try setting small, achievable goals that will help you make progress over time.

3. Celebrate your successes: It is important to celebrate your small wins and accomplishments. This can help you feel a sense of accomplishment and keep you motivated.

4. Be kind to yourself: It is easy to feel hard on yourself when you have a setback or make a mistake, but it is important to remember that everyone makes mistakes and that it is okay. Try to be kind and forgiving to yourself, and focus on what you can do to move forward.

5. Stay positive: It can be helpful to focus on the positive aspects of your diabetes management journey, such as the improvements you have made in your blood sugar control or the benefits of making healthy lifestyle choices.

By following these strategies, you can help maintain your motivation and stay on track with your diabetes reversal plan.

Chapter Eight

Tips for healthy grocery shopping with diabetes

Eating a healthy diet is important for everyone, but it can be especially important for people with diabetes to pay attention to the foods they eat and the quantities they consume. Here are some tips for healthy grocery shopping if you have diabetes:

Plan ahead: Make a list of the foods you need and stick to it. This can help you avoid impulse purchases of unhealthy foods.

Focus on whole, unprocessed foods: Choose foods that are minimally processed, such as fresh fruits and vegetables, whole grains, lean proteins, and healthy fats. These foods tend to be more nutrient-dense and can help you better manage your blood sugar levels.

Choose low-glycemic index foods: Foods with a low glycemic index (GI) are absorbed more slowly into the bloodstream, which can help prevent spikes in blood sugar levels. Examples of low-GI foods include whole grains, beans, and most vegetables.

Look for healthy fats: Choose foods that are rich in healthy fats, such as avocados, nuts, and olive oil. These fats can help you feel fuller longer and may also help improve blood sugar control.

Limit added sugars: Choose foods that are low in added sugars, such as those found in soda, sweetened beverages, and processed snacks. These types of sugars can contribute to high blood sugar levels.

Read labels: Pay attention to serving sizes and the number of carbohydrates per serving when shopping for packaged foods. This can help you make healthier choices and better manage your blood sugar levels.

Consider your medication: If you are taking medication to manage your diabetes, consider how different foods may affect your blood sugar levels. For example, some foods may interfere with the absorption of certain medications or may affect your blood sugar levels in unpredictable ways. It is important to talk to your healthcare provider about how different foods may affect your diabetes management plan.

Weekly Diabetes Meal Plan

Monday:

Breakfast: Overnight oats with chia seeds and fresh berries

Lunch: Grilled chicken and vegetable skewers with quinoa

Dinner: Slow cooker lentil soup with a side of roasted broccoli

Tuesday:

Breakfast: Avocado toast with scrambled eggs and cherry tomatoes

Lunch: Turkey and lettuce wraps with hummus and cucumber slices

Dinner: Grilled salmon with sweet potato wedges and roasted asparagus

Wednesday:

Breakfast: Greek yogurt with nuts, seeds, and fresh fruit

Lunch: Whole wheat pasta with grilled vegetables and a side salad

Dinner: Baked chicken with roasted vegetables and a quinoa pilaf

Thursday

Breakfast: Omelette with vegetables and a slice of whole grain toast

Lunch: Black bean and corn salad with a side of mixed fruit

Dinner: Grilled shrimp and zucchini noodles with a tomato basil sauce

Friday

Breakfast: Smoothie bowl with frozen fruit, yogurt, and nuts

Lunch: Turkey and avocado roll-ups with carrot sticks and hummus

Dinner: Slow cooker black bean and sweet potato chili with a side of brown rice

Saturday

Breakfast: Whole grain waffles with fresh berries and a drizzle of honey

Lunch: Grilled chicken Caesar salad with whole grain croutons

Dinner: Baked salmon with a quinoa and vegetable stir fry

Sunday

Breakfast: Scrambled eggs with spinach and whole grain toast

Lunch: Veggie wrap with hummus and a side of mixed fruit

Dinner: Slow cooker vegetarian chili with a side of cornbread

Conclusion

Achieving optimal health with diabetes requires a combination of proper medical care, a healthy lifestyle, and effective self-management. This includes working closely with a healthcare team to properly manage blood sugar levels, regularly monitoring blood sugar levels, and following a healthy diet and exercise plan. Additionally, it is important to follow a prescribed treatment plan, attend regular check-ups and screenings, and be aware of and manage any potential complications. By taking an active role in managing their diabetes, individuals with the condition can lead healthy and fulfilling lives.

Recap of the key points and strategies for reversing diabetes

Focus on nutrient-dense, whole foods: Choose ingredients that are rich in nutrients and low in added sugars and refined carbohydrates.

- Incorporate healthy fats: Healthy fats, such as those found in avocado, nuts, and olive oil, can help improve insulin sensitivity and lower blood sugar levels.

- Limit added sugars: Added sugars, such as those found in processed and packaged foods, can contribute to high blood sugar levels. Instead, opt for naturally sweet ingredients, such as fruit, to add flavor to recipes.

- Choose whole grains: Whole grains, such as quinoa, brown rice, and whole grain bread, are rich in fiber and can help improve blood sugar control.

- Include protein: Protein can help slow the absorption of carbohydrates and improve blood sugar control. Choose sources of protein, such as chicken, turkey, fish, beans, and tofu.

- Don't forget the vegetables: Vegetables are an important part of a healthy diet for diabetes management. Aim to include a variety of non-starchy vegetables, such as leafy greens, bell peppers, and broccoli, in your recipes.

- Use herbs and spices: Herbs and spices can add flavor to dishes without adding added sugars or sodium. Experiment with different combinations to find flavors that you enjoy.

Remember to always work with a healthcare provider or registered dietitian to determine the best diet and lifestyle strategies for your specific needs.